Multiple Sclerosis Nursing International Certification Examination

I0029982

A Step by step Guide on How To Prepare for

And

PASS the MSCN EXAM

Sample Questions included

ADAMA B. YANSANEH, BSN, RN, MSCN, CCM, CRNI, CCRN, CHC

Copyright: © 2016   Adama B. Yansaneh

All Rights reserved. No part of this book may be reproduced, transmitted, or distributed by any means or in any form without prior permission of the author, except in brief quotations or other non-commercial use allowed by copyright law.

This book is intended for educational and information purposes only. The book is mostly based on the Author's personal experience in preparing for the Multiple Sclerosis Certified Nurse exam. All efforts have been made to verify and clarify the information contained in this book. The Author takes no responsibilities for any omission, errors, or contrary information. The Author makes no expressed or implied warranty or guarantee. The reader assumes all risks in using or taking any advice from this publication.

CONTENTS

DEDICATION

This book is dedicated to people with Multiple Sclerosis and to all the nurses involved in their care, in various capacities, all around the world.

INTRODUCTION

A FOOL WITH A PLAN CAN OUTSMART A GENIUS WITH NO PLAN.
- Thomas Boone Pickens

When I was planning on taking the exam to become a Multiple Sclerosis Certified Nurse some time ago, I went to amazon.com and other related websites to find books and study guides for the Multiple Sclerosis Nursing International Certification Examination; I was able to find several books on Multiple Sclerosis, but I could not find books that were specific to the certification exam itself.

Nursing certification examinations are generally very challenging. Many well versed, very brilliant nurses have been known to fail these exams quite easily. One has to be well prepared, as well as have time-tested study strategies and techniques to challenge and pass nursing certification examinations of all kinds.

I am an experienced Registered Nurse, who has worked with patients across the lifespan, in various clinical settings. I make it a priority to learn as much as possible, to the point of getting certification, in almost every area of nursing I have been fortunate to work in. I am certified in Case Management, Infusion Nursing, Critical Care Nursing, and now, thank goodness, Multiple Sclerosis Nursing. For all the other certification examinations I have taken before, I could easily find several certification guide books online and at the local bookstores; that was not the case for the MSCN examination. I could have easily asked other Multiple Sclerosis Certified Nurses for guidance, but I decided to find the needed information on my own. I figured if I am successful in passing the examination by using resources that I found on my own, I will compile all the information for future use, for myself and for others who may need some personal guidance on what to do to prepare for this very important examination. In addition to the information on multiple sclerosis nursing exams study materials; I will share my own personal blueprint, tips, strategies and techniques I learnt, skills that helped me pass my Multiple Sclerosis Nursing Certification Examination.

<u>This book is a compilation of time-tested skills I have learnt and used over the years, to pass every single one of my nursing certification exams, each at the very first attempt.</u>

In addition to this book, I have also put together another book:-
"MSCN Exam Preparation: 150 Test Review Questions."
That book can be obtained and used as a separate unit, or it can be used as a companion to this book, for test practice and review tools, for the MSCN Exam.

I have had tremendous success and benefits from using the test taking skills I have gathered and recorded in these books. I sincerely hope my readers will find both books as invaluable tools to add to their arsenal of study materials for this very important certification exam.

Adama B Yansaneh, BSN, RN, MSCN, CCM, CRNI, CCRN, CHC

Contact information: **<u>adayans@gmail.com</u>** or **info@elitecarecorp.com**

CHAPTER ONE

FIRST THINGS FIRST

For anyone preparing to take the MSCN exam, do re-examine your learning style and study habits. Figure out what has worked well for you in past nursing examinations. Be honest with yourself about where you think you may need to make some improvements. Be very self-motivated, aspire to get your certification because you desire to improve your clinical knowledge, not just because your employer requires that you do so. Be a life-long learner. Be willing to study hard.

For the MSCN and every other certification exams, learn as much content as possible, but focus mostly on the areas of the exam that have the highest weighted percentage scores. Make yourself very familiar with the blueprint of the exam and use it as a guide to know which areas you need to focus on the most during your studies.

When planning to take any certification exam, you of course find out who prepares or administers the exam, find out what the exam schedule is and how much the exam will cost, among other things. As you do all of that, be sure to make yourself very familiar with the BLUEPRINT of the certification exam itself. As per information from their website, the MSCN exam is prepared by the Multiple Sclerosis Nursing International Certification Board (MSNICB) with assistance and advice from Professional Testing Corporation (PTC). Website: ptcny.com

Visit the website of Multiple Sclerosis Nurses International Certification Board (MSNICB)

On the news tracker, the exam schedule dates are highlighted; it is also listed in the Main Menu.

The Main Menu on the website has other itemized information links, each of which is worth reviewing thoroughly.

Click on MSCN Certification Guidelines and download the

MSNICB HANDBOOK.

Read the eligibility requirements, the exam cost, then start looking at the Blue print of the exam. On the Main Menu, click on the area labeled "Resources list" for information on the textbook "Nursing Practice in MS: A Core Curriculum." I started my studies for the MSCN exam with reading this book, back to back. The book has 10 Case Studies and 50 Practice Questions that are worth reviewing. I bought my copy of this book at a much lower price on Amazon Kindle.

When I first visited the MSNICB website, just as an aside, I clicked on the list of "Passing Candidates" on the Menu section. I envisioned my name being on that list someday after I take and pass the MSCN exam. I kept that image vivid and engrained in my head all through my studies for the MSCN exam. I formed a mental picture of my name with the credentials: "Adama Yansaneh, BSN, RN, MSCN."

Still on the website, I clicked on the section labeled "Affiliates" to be redirected to other very important links. A click on the links will direct one to a lot of MS learning resources. From here, reading materials, On Demand Videos and so on can be found at the web pages of The International Organization of Multiple Sclerosis Nurses (IOMSN) and the Consortium of Multiple Sclerosis Centers (CMSC). You will certainly learn a lot about MS from the resources on all of these websites.

CHAPTER TWO

Blueprint of the Multiple Sclerosis Nursing International Certification Examination

The Multiple Sclerosis Nursing International Certification Examinations has a maximum of 150 questions. The testing time is 2.5 hours.According to the MSNICB Exam Handbook, the test grades are weighted as follows:

CONCEPTS UNDERLYING CLINICAL PRACTICE: 23%
ASSESSMENT AND INTERVENTION FOR CLINICAL
PRACTICE   42%
ADVOCACY   10%
EDUCATION   17%
RESEARCH   8%

"ASSESSMENT AND INTERVENTION for CLINICAL PRACTICE" has the highest weighted area. This area is allotted a warping 42%, almost half of the entire exam grade. To me, this meant that I had to allot most of my study time to the thorough understanding of the subject matter, the concepts/ content in this particular area. I had to know the information in this area, "like the back of my hand." I will try to know the information here "in my sleep," I thought to myself. I must know the information here, from the basic to the complex, to the point that I can simplify the content in my own words, well enough to be able to figuratively explain it well for any lay person to understand, I said to myself.
EXAM STUDY STRATEGY # 1: For my study purposes, I re-arranged the various areas of the exam weighted percentages, so the numbers will be highlighted from highest to lowest:

ASSESSMENT AND INTERVENTION FOR CLINICAL
PRACTICE: 42%
CONCEPTS UNDERLYING CLINICAL PRACTICE: 23%
EDUCATION: 17%

ADVOCACY: 10%
RESEARCH: 8%

In the handbook, right below the listed weighted numbers, an outline and summary of the topics covered in the various areas are listed.

FYI: The Exam handbook has five practice questions that are worth answering

After I had made myself familiar with what was required to take the exam, I filled out the application form, chose an exam date and paid the examination fee of $300.00 to PTC: Professional Testing Corporation right away. I got an exam date, I had an exam schedule, I had now incurred a cost of $300.00; everything became real for me. I had paid $300.00 to the PTC testing center; this was now a full commitment for me. I became even more determined to study hard, so I can pass the MSCN exam at the very first attempt. I did not want to forfeit my hard earned $300.00 for any reason whatsoever. My understanding is that, if one does not take the exam, a partial refund of $50.00 or so, will be given back, provided a request is submitted in writing, up to 30 days after the date of the test. That still meant a forfeiture of some of my money; I did not want that to happen at all. Money aside, though, above all else, I really actually just wanted to get my MSCN certification. So, I said to myself "Adama, Buckle up, it is time to study; study very hard, leave no stone unturned, do the utmost best, pass the MSCN exam at the very first attempt. So Help Me God!"

Well, there is an old African saying:

"When you ask God to help you, God will say: "help yourself first"

The meaning of the saying is that regardless of one's faith in God, one must have self-initiative. One must work hard to achieve desired goals. One must not just wait to have things happen by chance or by luck.

In other words, it simply means "God helps those who help themselves"

I was willing to study hard, prepare well, so I can pass the Multiple Sclerosis Nursing International Certification Examination at my very first attempt. I put the exam date on my mobile phone calendar. I posted paper copies of the exam schedule on the refrigerator and other areas in my house. I made sure I could see the exam information in some very prominent areas in my home. I was now much more focused, very mentally and physically prepared, ready to study intensively and extensively, leave no stone unturned, give it my all, to pass the exam at just one attempt. I had strategic study plans and test taking techniques in place, to give me the best chance of reaching my goal, to become certified at my set date and deadline.

I used the blue print of the exam, as outlined in the MSNICB handbook, as my guide during my studies for the exam. I had the exam handbook at my side at all times. I referred to the exam content/ the exam blue print very often during my study periods. I assigned specific number of days to cover each individual section or area thoroughly, so as to enhance my ability to study and comprehend content material outlined in the MSNICB exam handbook.

CHAPTER THREE

The General "Blueprint" for Nursing Certification Exams

The blueprint, the framework, the backbone for critical thinking competency for nurses is the NURSING PROCESS. Phases of the nursing process are Assessment, Analyses/Nursing Diagnosis, Planning, Implementation, and Evaluation. The Nursing Process is utilized to critically think and implement nursing interventions to maximize patient outcomes. Phases of the Nursing Process are included in the Multiple Sclerosis Nursing International Certification Exam, with "Assessment and Intervention for Clinical Practice" being the areas of highest concentration.

Bloom's Taxonomy of learning namely: Knowledge, Comprehension, Application, Analysis, Synthesis, and evaluation are levels of cognition nursing exams candidates must be familiar with. Knowledge is at the lowest level of Blooms Cognitive Taxonomy; analysis, synthesis and evaluation are at the highest levels.

Nursing examinations test the nurse's ability to utilize knowledge; to comprehend, implement, synthesize and evaluate situations, in order to maximize patient outcomes. The nurse must be able to apply previously learnt information in new situations to make competent and safe clinical judgments and decisions.

The nurse has to have knowledge and comprehension of required content in order to be able to recall, define, recognize and select relevant clinical information and actions to implement at the appropriate times. The nurse must be able to comprehend, understand, explain, present, interpret and distinguish between different patient situations and case scenarios in order to have safe patient outcomes. As an exam candidate, you must comprehend the required content and information well, in order to enhance your ability to make critical application decisions in the right circumstance, at the right time.

Application of information learnt is implemented in new situations to problem solve. Application type questions usually require one to use a previously learnt knowledge to problem solve or modify new situations to maximize or improve patient outcomes.

In Analyses type questions, one has to be able to interpret data, distinguish between common relationships and situations. One must examine, evaluate and analyze information for correctness, then synthesize the data, using critical thinking, to intervene appropriately and safely in new or different patient situations.

The nurse must be able to use critical thinking skills to put ideas together, to arrive at new conclusions. The nurse has to critically Analyze, Synthesize, and Evaluate clinical situations, to arrive at the best decisions, best judgments that are clinically safe and appropriate for the patient.

The nurse has to Analyze, differentiate, and evaluate issues in new or different situations. The nurse has to synthesize information by utilizing high critical thinking skills to problem solve.

Overall, it is worth repeating that one has to have knowledge and understanding of required content, then build upon previously learnt knowledge to correctly answer the higher levels application, analysis and evaluations questions.

In looking further at Blooms Taxonomy, one can see that the lower levels of cognition tests one's basic ability to recall and recognize information.

Sample stem questions here have words like (What, Which, When, How many, which one and so on.) They are meant to test one's ability to recall or recognize relevant content.

Sample Question:

Approximately what percentage of patients with MS have the Relapsing-remitting form of the disease?

    A: 50%
    B: 85%
    C: 25%
    D: 75%

The correct answer is- B: 85%. This answer is just a recall of previously learnt information.Testing of ones understanding type questions may start with Stems or Keywords like: Select, Clarify, Explain, Choose, Which, What and so on.

Sample Question:

Which of the following medications is used to possibly manage the frequency of relapses in MS?

    A: Baclofen
    B: Ampyra
    C: Glatiramer Acetate
    D: Modafinil

The correct answer is- C: Glatiramer Acetate. The nurse uses his/her understanding of medication classes and types to answer this question.
An example of a comprehension type question may be seen in situations such as patient education. Keywords may include words like:

Compare, Contrast, Explain, Teach, Translate, Show, Name a few and so on. Question formats, for example, may ask one to state facts, show which is the best answer and so on. The nurse, therefore, has to comprehend facts and information in order to provide effective patient teaching. The nurse has to show understanding of facts in this type of questions.

EXAMPLE:

A nurse is providing medication teaching to a Multiple Sclerosis patient who has just found out that she is pregnant. The patient was originally on Tecfidera, an oral disease-modifying agent, but the physician has changed her medication to Copaxone injections. The patient tells the nurse that she prefers oral medications to injectable agents.

The nurse when teaching about the relevant disease -modifying agents will tell this patient that:

> A: Tecfidera is easier and better to take during pregnancy because it does not require any injections to the abdomen.
> B: Copaxone is a pregnancy category-B drug and is therefore comparably less risky in pregnancy than Tecfidera.
> C: Tecfidera is an oral medication and has no risk on the growing fetus
> D: Copaxone is an injectable disease-modifying agent that should never be used in pregnancy.

The correct Answer is B: The nurse understands drug safety/ risks in pregnancy. The Nurse uses her understanding of FDA pregnancy category risk of drugs for patient teaching in this situation.

Application type questions require the nurse to "apply" knowledge she already has to a given situation, to provide relevant, safe nursing care. The nurse has to use his/her knowledge to prioritize care.

Sample Keywords here Include:
(Choose, Identify, Apply, First, Least, Last and so on.)

EXAMPLE: You are performing a nursing assessment on a patient with advanced MS. The daughter tells you that the patient has had some recent fevers, occasional shortness of breath, constipation and pressure ulcers, among other things. Which of the following will you do first?

A: Assess vital signs, including respiratory system.
B: Assess bowel sounds and bowel patterns.
C: Check patient's skin including the pressure ulcer site.
D: Check patient's dietary and feeding patterns

The correct Answer is: A

All of the stated issues are important but the ABCs, for example, take precedence over the others.

Using the same patient as in the previous situation, the nurse could use her knowledge of advanced MS and possible patient complications of the disease at this stage, to implement a plan of care and nursing interventions for the patient. The nurse will analyze this situation and realize that swallowing problems, pressure ulcers, contractures are all issues that can arise with MS at the advanced stages of the disease. The nurse will analyze and evaluate data, then determine what the most appropriate nursing actions will be to problem solve in various patient situations.

Analyses questions could require the nurse to identify problems, outcomes, distinguish between situations and so on. When planning for required nursing actions, the nurse could make inferences, draw conclusions, identify causes, reasons from given information to support facts and provide safe care.

Keywords at the Analyses level may include:
Analyze, Distinguish, List, and Examine, to name a few.

Regardless of which step or theory the Stem or Question is based on, the nurse, as the caregiver, has to eventually evaluate situations and make good clinical judgments, based on valid, evidence-based criteria.

With the blueprint of the Multiple Sclerosis Nursing International Certification Examination in mind and taking into consideration the general blueprint of nursing certification exams, I then moved on to my next step, namely: putting together all the materials and resources I needed to study and prepare for my certification exam.

CHAPTER FOUR

Books that I used to study for the Multiple Sclerosis Nursing Certification exam

The following are among some of the books I read to prepare for the exam.

1: Nursing Practice in Multiple Sclerosis: A Core Curriculum
Third Edition.
Authors: June Halper, MSN, APN-C, MSCN, FAAN
Colleen Harris, MN, NP, MSCN
FYI: This book has Case Studies in Chapter 21 and chapter 22 has 50 Personal review questions. I read the entire book including the Appendices B, C, D, and E, then I answered the Personal Review and Case study questions.

FYI: A new edition/A fourth edition of this book is available, September 2016

Note: If I am press for time and money and can afford to get only one book, this book will be the one I will choose to get. This, of course, is just my personal opinion. There is no guarantee that reading this book or any of the others mentioned here will secure one's success in the MSCN exam.

2: Comprehensive Nursing Care in Multiple Sclerosis
Third Edition
June Halper, MSN, APN-C, FAAN, MSCN
Nancy Joyce Holland, EdD, RN, MSCN

3: Multiple Sclerosis from Both Side of the Desk
Author: Vincent F. Macaluso, MD

FYI: Dr. Macaluso is a physician who was diagnosed with MS while he was in medical school.

4: Multiple Sclerosis: Clinician's Guide to Diagnosis and Treatment
  Edited by: Gary Birnbaum, MD

5: Multiple Sclerosis for Dummies
  Authors: Rosalind Kalb, Ph.D., Barbara Giesser, MD, and
Kathleen Costello, ANP-BC

I love reading the "DUMMIES" series books.
As the books /series claim, they are "Making Everything Easier"
In the books for Dummies Series subject matters/concepts are
explained in a much more simple and memorable way, most times
with humor and picture illustrations.
For me personally, when ideas are taught, explained with pictures,
or humor, I tend to remember the concepts and information
better.
I can visualize the concepts or ideas well; my brain can recall such
information much more easily.

6: 100 Questions & Answers about Multiple Sclerosis.
  Second Edition.
  William A. Sheremata, MD, FRCPC, FACP

  I got this book later after I had already taken and passed the
MSCN exam. If I had this book in my possession beforehand, I
would have used it in the following manner. I would have read this
book to understand most of the 100 questions and answers. After
making myself familiar with the content provided, I would have
put the book aside for a while, go on to read my other MS books,
then re-visit this book at a later time, to see if I could successfully
answer as many of the questions as possible. In other words, I
would have used this book mostly as part of my "Practice and
Review Question and Answer Sessions."

CHAPTER FIVE

Websites that I personally found helpful for the exam

1: <u>MSNICB.ORG</u> : This is the website of the Multiple Sclerosis Nurses International Certification Board.

The MSNICB website is the first place to visit to get all the necessary information one needs to know about the MSCN examination itself. The website has guidelines, information on fees, the exams, resources and a lot of other very useful information. I personally visited and reviewed every link listed in the Main Menu section of the website. I found the MSCNIB website to be very thorough and helpful.

2: <u>IOMSN.ORG</u> : This is the website of the International Organization of Multiple Sclerosis Nurses.

You don't have to be a member to access or benefit from this website. There are lots of good education materials, links to articles, journals, audiovisual materials and other MS resources on this site. This website has a section labeled "Reference Materials." I clicked on every one of the links in the reference section and reviewed as much of the listed information as I could.
 I downloaded the 100 page E-book:
NURSE'S QUICK reference: CARING FOR PATIENTS WITH MULTIPLE SCLEROSIS
 By Anthony Ayag, RN, MSCN.

This is a great reference tool, a really good piece of work! I read this reference book back to back, at least twice.
I would like to take this opportunity to sincerely thank
Anthony Ayag, RN, MSCN, the author of this E-book!

Thank You Anthony!

3: <u>mscare.org</u> cMSc The Consortium of Multiple Sclerosis Centers website is another great site that has lots of links, informative articles on MS, current medications, On Demand Webinars and so on.

4: <u>msviews.org</u> this is another great site for MS patients, their caregivers and health care providers combined.

There are blogs, videos, articles and a lot of great learning information tools on this website. Links to the various MS medications websites are also listed in the information section on the toolbar of the website.

I have the utmost respect, gratitude and admiration for Stuart Schlossman, President, and Founder of MS Views and News.

Thank You, Stuart!

5: <u>NationalMSsociety.org</u> : This is another one stop center for videos, PDFs and other learning tools about MS. Learn about MS 101 on this site.

In my bid to absolutely make sure I thoroughly understood the pathophysiology, the etiology, the treatment and nursing care of patients with MS, to the very best of my ability, to make sure I left no stone unturned for the MSCN exam, I also did the following:

A: I viewed Khan Academy videos both on their website and on YouTube.

B: I watched Kaplan videos about Multiple Sclerosis on YouTube: presented by Dr. Conrad Fischer, Residency Program Director at Brook dale University Center, NY.

When one listens to Dr. Fischer teach anything, the ideas just stay in one's memory somehow. His teaching style is remarkable and memorable. Dr. Conrad Fischer is funny and just really good at what he does! Thank you, Dr. Fischer!

C: I watched a video presentation: "Multiple Sclerosis: Signs, Symptoms, and Treatment," a talk given by Christina Johnston, DO, Neurologist at Lakeshore Partners, Holland, Michigan
 You can find her video on YouTube too.
Thank you, Dr. Johnston!

D: I also watched the Multiple Sclerosis-Crash! Medical Review Series on YouTube.

There are many more helpful websites not named in this book. The ones mentioned here are suggestions for some of the resources I used and found beneficial for the MSCN Exam. One does not have to read so many books and journals; one does not have to visit so many websites to study for or pass this exam. One can choose to use all, or just a combination of some of the aforementioned resources, since the information tends to be repeated from one area to the other.

I visited several MS websites, watched several YouTube videos, read a combination of books on MS (both E-books and paper books.) In addition to reading quite a few books on MS, I also watched several online videos, presented by health care experts and patients alike. I tried to cover all my bases for this exam. I was prepared, for as much as my personal and work schedules would permit. I immersed myself, full-fledged, into studying for the exam.

When once I had made the decision and personal commitment to take the Multiple Sclerosis Nursing International Certification Exam, I became determined to give it my all. I was going to use every available study resource I had access to, in order to make sure I accomplish my goal of passing the exam at my very first attempt. It is true I did not want to have my $300.00 go in vain, money aside, though; I really just wanted to get my MSCN credentials. I strive to do all I can to continue to improve my knowledge of Multiple Sclerosis nursing care.

Personally, I believe that achieving the MSCN credential is invaluable for nurses who work with Multiple Sclerosis patients.

CHAPTER SIX

Background facts to note when studying for certification exams

As you start your studies for this exam, please always be aware of the following important facts:

Nurses in all clinical settings are required and expected to use critical thinking skills.

The ability to have critical thinking skills is a must for every nurse.

Nurses are expected to have good clinical judgment and competent critical decisions making skills.

Nurses, as health care professionals, are held to very high standards.

Nurses must strive to promote and protect patients' rights.

Nurses must strive to protect the health and safety of patients.

The patient is the focus; the patient is the central person in the realm of nursing and health care.

Nurses are patient advocates.

Nursing practice must be supported by current evidence-based research.

Nurses as patient advocates and care providers play very important roles in Multiple Sclerosis Research.

The Multiple Sclerosis Certified Nurse has to have command of common knowledge of Multiple Sclerosis disease.

The Multiple Sclerosis Certified Nurse has to have critical knowledge and critical thinking skills to function safely and effectively when providing care for Multiple Sclerosis patients.

Remember these important facts as you answer every one of the questions in the certification exam setting. You are indirectly held accountable for every one of these standards, as you answer every nursing certification exam test question. It is important to not lose sight of these facts, not only during this exam, but in every clinical setting, for as long as one is a practicing nursing professional.

CHAPTER SEVEN

My Personal Study Pattern and Study Tips for the Exam

Days Allocated for studying: 45 DAYS
I usually prefer to set 90 days of study time, whenever possible. Please, choose how much time period will work best for you personally.

For me, it is usually 45 to 90 days from study prep. time to exam day. For this exam, I read books, journals and website information. I watched online videos and did something related to studying for the exam on almost every one of the 45 days I had set aside to prepare for the exam.

I started my studying for the exam by reading the books and items listed on the MSNICB and IOMSN Websites. I figured the exam is made and set by them, they must know more about relevant resources for the exam, I thought. I read the two resources listed below first.

1: Multiple Sclerosis: A core Curriculum
2: Nurse's Quick reference: Caring for Patients with Multiple Sclerosis

I usually study in 20 to 30 minutes increment at a time, taking frequent breaks, in between. I kept the MSNICB Exam Handbook at my side as I read books, referred to it frequently, paying more attention to core topics that are mentioned in the exam blueprint. I focused more intensely on the content areas that have the highest percentage weight, as per the MSNICB exam handbook, namely: Assessment and Interventions for Clinical practice: 42%; Concepts Underlying Clinical Practice: 23%, Education: 17%, Advocacy: 10%, Research: 8%)

The exam handbook, the syllabus/content outline was at my side at all times during my studies, I referred to the handbook frequently, just to make sure I had all the relevant content areas covered. I used the" syllabus "of the handbook to guide me as I studied for the exam. I made myself familiar with every listed content, line by line, but as stated previously, I did focus more intensely on the highest weighted percentage grade areas.

I started the online video watching sessions with the video presented by Dr. Christina Johnston. This video talks about Multiple Sclerosis from definitions, diagnosis, signs & symptoms and treatment. After watching that video, I went on to watch other online videos presentations by physicians like Dr. Conrad Fischer.

The National MS Society website has easy to understand videos for patients and caregivers alike. I watched several of their website and YouTube videos.

I watched multiple sclerosis videos on websites of Khan Academy, MS Views and News and other MS related websites. As I read books, visited websites and watched online videos, I made relevant notes, Mnemonics, and Acronyms. I also formulated and answered several personal review/practice questions, all in an effort to enhance my comprehension and retention of relevant study subject matter.

I also USED the PQRST acronym as a study tool in the following ways:

P: Previewed the chapters or materials briefly, for few minutes, scanning, looking at the headings, subheadings, reading the introductions and summaries, to know what each chapter was talking about. I payed specific attention to areas in the chapters that are related to the exam Blueprint.

Q: Questioned what the main point of a chapter was about. Created questions about the important points, kept those questions in mind during my readings. The questions were geared towards

21

understanding the important concepts outlined in the Exam Handbook. I paraphrased important points and wrote them down at the edge of the textbooks or on index cards.

R: Read in a more focused and active manner, relating the information in the reading to the questions I had formulated earlier. Recited the main points in my own words repeatedly, so as to comprehend the information even better.

S: Summarized the main ideas in my own words and read them out to myself. I wrote short notes, made Acronyms and Mnemonics to help me comprehend the topics even better.

T: Tested myself by answering the questions I had created earlier. I made sure I could answer the questions while the book was closed, then opened the book to verify my answers. I repeated the process over and over until I could answer the questions without looking at the relevant areas in the books.

As nurses, we know PQRST is an acronym used in nursing assessment of patients in pain. It can stand for Pain, Quality, Radiates, Severity, and Time. In ECG rhythm interpretations, it can stand for the various parts of the electrical waveforms: P wave, QRS complex, and the ST segment.

I used the PQRST method to review my notes, the main ideas, and the various videos and so on, to commit relevant information to my long term memory. To enhance my comprehension during my studies, I verbalized the main ideas to myself, in my own words. I did numerous reviews of the main ideas about MS in my study materials, to help me understand and retain the relevant information needed for the exam.

Below are sample mnemonics I made to help me remember some current Multiple Sclerosis Medications. I had them listed from oral, injectable to intravenous in the following manner:

ORAL: Tecfidera, Aubagio, Gilenya ———(**TAG**)

INJECTIONS: Betaseron, Extavia, Copaxone, Rebif, Avonex, Plegridy — **(BE CRAP)**

INTRAVENOUS: Novantrone, Lemtrada, Tysabri
(NO LONE TIME) or **(NO LOVE TIME)**

The more outrageous the story, acronym or mnemonic, the better I can recall the information. That last mnemonic is outrageous for sure because I do believe we all have to make time for love in our everyday lives.
On the day of the exam, when I received the scratch paper, I did the "BRAIN DUMP" right away. I wrote: TAG, BE CRAP, NO LOVE TIME, Neuron, Axon, myelin dendrite, white matter, oligodendrocytes, etc. on the scratch paper before I even started taking the exam. I had made up ways to connect these words and ideas in my head. With the "Brain Dump" they were all on the scratch paper as my reference tool, just in case, for some unexplained reason, I needed something to trigger my memory during the exam.

When studying medications, I mostly study them by classifications and mechanism of action. I try to remember important variations among medication groups. I try to learn about the most common and the most serious effects. I pay special attention to relevant patient safety issues associated with the various medication classes.

Examples of some interferons: Betaseron, Avonex, Rebif, Extavia **(BARE)** for acronym.
Know side effects to monitor for e.g. flu-like symptoms in the interferon, injection site reactions and so on.

Know the most serious safety concern for each group of drugs e.g. Tysabri (PML) Progressive multifocal Leukoencephalopathy. PML in Tysabri and also in Tecfidera

John Cunningham virus (The JC Virus). (Lab work) Virus related to PML

Know safety monitoring parameters, know the labs to monitor for different medication classifications.
Example: Complete blood count, liver enzymes with the Interferons and oral MS medications.

In the case of child-bearing age females, pregnancy risk may be a concern. Know which medications are comparably, "safer" for childbearing MS patients e.g.: COPAXONE VS Tecfidera.

Basically, know the most common Multiple Sclerosis medications. Understand risks, patient safety issues that may arise with each of them. Know what the nurse can do in such cases to prevent problems and promote safety in different patient situations.

Do as many practice questions as you can. The Professional Testing Corporation has practice questions one can review before the exams.
At this time, the cost is $50.00 for 50 questions. I believe a lot of people will find these website practice questions very helpful. I did not use the service because I had formulated several review/practice questions of my own.

Practicing Review Questions can be very helpful for this exam. They help one understand and retain important concepts even better. They give the MSCN candidate an idea of what the exam questions may look like. Questions from practice exams may sometimes show up in actual examinations, but the wording or format maybe different. It is therefore helpful to do as many practice questions as possible to prepare for certification exams. If you can afford it, take the online practice test, for more review and practice before the actual exam day.

I know that different people have different learning styles, Use whatever learning style works best for you. I try to use a combination of different learning styles to stimulate the various areas of my brain; I retain various content material better that way. The Visual, Aural, Verbal, Physical, Social, Solitary, Logical, I combine as many of these learning styles as I can, so as to challenge my brain to retain learning materials even more.

When I study for exams, in my head, I try to create ridiculous, outrageous, humorous stories about important concepts. I can recall relevant information much more easily this way, whenever the need arises. I try to be more active and engaged in my learning, in whatever way I can.

Repetition of the learning materials in various forms help me commit the ideas to my Long Term memory. I use kinesthetic, visual, auditory all the learning styles combined when I am studying materials for examinations.

Personally, the idea of repetition of important concepts help me to remember and learn better when I study for exams. I take time to access and use as many resources as I can, review and study as much relevant information as I can, to help enhance my comprehension and retention of important exam subject matter.

I had my study information repeated in various formats, by various sets of experts, to the point that my brain could visualize the concepts and ideas much more easily, to be recalled "On Demand!" at the Testing Center, on the day of my exam.
For the MSCN exam, I watched presentations given by Nurses, by Physicians and by some MS patients themselves. I tried to learn more about Multiple Sclerosis from every credible, evidence-based resource I could find.

My personal Mantra for preparing for the MSCN and other nursing certification exams:

Study, Study, Study
Practice, Practice, Practice
Over study subject content
Use Critical Thinking
Over practice sample test questions.

Remember test taking tips.
Leave no stone unturned!

CHAPTER EIGHT

More Study tips for Nursing Certification Exams

First the Basics:
Nursing Certification Exams Require Critical Thinking and Good Clinical Judgment.

Choose your core study materials, your core resources and use them well. If you think you may be overwhelmed by too much information, choose to use only the resources that will work best for you personally.

.

I have mentioned some study resources in this book; you don't have to use all of them. Please use what will work best for you.

Know what your specific test taking problems are and try to work on improving those issues.

Have your family on board.
Have a good support system, whenever possible.

Take care of yourself. Have healthy meals, have a good exercise plan.

As you study for this exam, take small breaks, eat healthy meals, and take good care of yourself.

As you prepare to take this exam, have good time management system.

Remember: **Know the BLUEPRINT of the EXAM.** As you prepare for this exam, know what content areas the exam is focused on. Go to the MSNICB, print or download the Handbook and use it as a guide. Take into account the weighted percentage grade offered to each content area. You may not learn all the content, but learn as much as possible the information in the area that is allotted the highest weighted grade. Study as much as you can but, if you have very limited time to study, then focus more on the areas that have the highest awarded percentage grade.

During your studies, **have the MSNICB exam HANDBOOK HANDY** for referral to the exam blueprint. **Focus, focus, focus.**

The questions in the exam are not isolated by content or framework, but if one studies the content and framework of the exam very well, this will increase the chances of comprehending the content well enough to be able to apply knowledge learnt to resolve complex patient issues presented in the actual exam.
Learn the content well enough to comprehend key concepts. Increase your ability to use critical thinking skills to apply knowledge learnt to questions presented in the exam setting.
Learn, understand, and comprehend content. Have the knowledge, comprehend it enough to be able to apply, analyze and synthesize information in different clinical patient situations.
Comprehend content enough to be able to analyze, synthesize, evaluate, put ideas together to arrive at new judgments, new conclusions that are clinically safe and appropriate for the patient.

Remember to schedule your exam date even before you start your studies. Print the information from the website and post two or more copies somewhere very visible, so you can see the copies every day.
Hold yourself accountable to studying effectively to your set test date.

Keep your focus on the "EXAM ZONE" for the weeks or months you have set aside for this exam.
Know as much content material as you can, learn subject content very well so you reduce your chances of getting "zapped" by distractors in the actual exam questions on your test date.

Choose a quiet place for your studies.

For the period of time that you are preparing for the exam, immerse yourself in your studies. Do so for as much as you can when you are preparing to take the MSCN exam. If you can, study some every day, no matter how little. Your study period is not for a life time, it will go by fast, so dedicate your time an energy to studying effectively for your certification exam.

Study as much as you can for that allotted time that you have set aside for this exam.

Do as many Practice Questions as you can before the exam day. Comprehend; understand what is asked in the questions. Be able to comprehend, analyze and evaluate key situations presented in the questions.

Prepare well, give yourself the best shot to pass your certification exam at your very self attempt!

Be self-motivated!

Study, Study, Study

CHAPTER NINE

Test Taking Tips For Nursing Certification Exams

1: The NURSING PROCESS: When I am taking nursing exams of any kind, I always have the Nursing Process at the back of my mind.

If applicable, know what part of the nursing process is in individual questions: Assessment, Diagnosis, Planning/Outcomes, Implementation and Evaluation.

If the stem of the question is asking an Assessment related issue, for example, then eliminate the answers that are not talking about assessment. If it is an assessment question, try to make sure the assessment action matches what the question is asking.

Match the answer to what is stated in the question: For example, if the question is asking for an assessment of a situation, then the answer choice that is a nursing intervention may not be the correct one.

Match the part of the nursing process in the question to your choice of the answer option.

Whenever applicable, look at a question and figure out what part of the Nursing Process the question is based on. This will help guide you to choose the correct answer choice, based on the nursing process and the nursing action the question is looking for.
Be sure the option you choose is the most patient-centered; be sure it is the answer option that offers the best patient outcome in the presented scenario.

2: Don't forget MASLOW's Hierarchy of Needs namely: Physiologic/Biologic needs, Safety needs, Love and Belonging needs, Esteem needs and Self-Actualization.
Biologic/Physiologic needs come before safety, love, esteem and self-actualization needs.

When a question is stating various nursing interventions as choices, the answer choice that prioritizes the patient's Physiologic need is likely to be more correct than the one that is based on Self-Actualization or needs. Think MASLOW, think "Priority" when looking at the answer choices.

Choose the answer choice that is the most priority and safe solution in the presented scenario.

Keywords like: Most Important, Highest Priority, First, Last, Least, Essential, Immediate, Initial, First, Best and so on. may be some clues in these areas.

When more than one answer choice is correct, prioritize. Choose the answer option that best addresses the immediate need, the priority need of the patient, at that specific time, in that specific situation or case scenario.

3: The ABCs in Nursing Care: Nursing priority of patient care is very important. In the ABCs of Airway, Breathing, and Circulation concept, airway problems are addressed first.
If the ABCD Acronym means: Assessment, Basic Vitals, Charting, and Drugs, then one focuses on the "Assessment" which could include basic vital signs of the patient.

Choose the answer that has the Highest Priority.
Patient safety and best outcomes must take precedence during nursing care. Emergency patient situations always take precedence over other nonemergency issues.

4: THERAPEUTIC COMMUNICATIONS Principles: Reflection, Clarification, Silence, Confirmation, Summarization,

Facilitation, Restating are some of the techniques used when communicating with patients and families.

Example: In Restating, a Patient might say the following:

Patient: "I can't sleep, my mind keeps wondering."

Nurse: "You have trouble sleeping."

Nurses must use therapeutic responses that will acknowledge and validate what the patient is feeling. Unless there is a medical emergency, it is important to validate the patient's feeling first before doing other non-emergency nursing interventions. Whenever necessary or indicated, validate the feelings of the subject stated in the question.

Nursing actions that give allowance to patients to verbalize their feelings are preferable. Use open communication, open-ended questions. Allow the patient/client to have time or chance to think. Let the client/patient feel that he or she is listened to.

Use therapeutic responses that acknowledge and validate patient's feelings and needs. It is important to validate patient's feeling, especially so in test situations where you have more than one correct therapeutic response option.

5: Age, Sex, time frame, can all be significant pointers to important leads in nursing exam questions. They may show an expected or unexpected finding in a particular group of people at a particular time. Remember **Erikson's Stages of Psychosocial Development**. Align the psychosocial needs of the patient's age group when an age is given in a question. Ask if the psychosocial response matches the age or actions in the answer choice?

6: Documentation: Remember that nursing actions must be documented accordingly. Drug administration must be documented using the five/six rights: **Right Patient, Right Drug,**

Right Dose, Right Route, Right Time, Right Documentation and Right Situation.

7: Delegation: Delegate stable patients only. Delegate appropriately. Delegate Safely. Delegate the right task, under the right circumstance, to the right person. Give the right directions, supervise in the right manner and evaluate in the right way after the task is performed. Evaluate to make sure the delegated task was performed accurately; in a timely manner and that the client's needs were met. Make sure the person you are delegating to is well qualified, well trained to perform the task you are delegating. Do not delegate to unqualified personnel.

8: Physician Notification: It may sound simple, but know when to notify the physician. In the case of stable patients, usually, questions that have nursing actions are more correct than ones that contain the words "Notify the physician"

9: Know that your expertise and knowledge is very crucial in providing appropriate patient teaching.

Example: A question that requires the nurse to do some more teaching may go like this:

"A 24-year-old newly diagnosed Multiple Sclerosis patient has just been placed on Glatiramer Acetate, 40 mg injection. Which statement (s) made by the client indicate (s) a need for further teaching?

   A: I must space my injections about every 48 hours
   B: I must inject myself three times a week
   C: I must massage the injection site right after injecting, to make sure the medicine works well.
   D: I must keep an eye on my injection sites for skin reactions.

C is the correct answer.

Here the nurse knows massaging the injection site right after administering Copaxone injection is not a recommended practice or technique:
The patient must avoid massaging the injection site on the day of the injection.

Remember, before patient teaching; confirm that the patient is motivated and ready for learning.

10: Understand **exams questions well. Read the question and make sure you know what the question is asking before you choose your answer from the given options.**

Understand what the question wants you to know, or wants you to do the MOST.
Distinguish the relevant facts from the distractors in the question.
Look at the parts of the question. Read the question well; understand what the question is asking.
Know the scenario/the case presented.
When ever possible ask yourself the following questions:
What are the issues presented in the question?
What is the problem in the presented scenario?
What is the problem related to?
Is the problem a sign/symptom of a disease?
Is it a side effect of a drug?
Is it about a behavior?
Who is presented in the case? Who is the focus of the question?
What is happening to that person?
What is the nursing action required?
Is the nursing action related to a specific part of the nursing process?
Is it about patient priority?
Is it about patient safety issues?
Understand what the question is asking. Do not read into or over analyze test questions.

11: Identify WHO or WHAT the question is actually focused on.

The focus of some of the questions may be friends, relatives, significant others or spouses of patients. Know who the focus of the question is.

12: In an exam question, there is the part that has the correct response, then there are the other choices that may not be correct for one particular question, but may be appropriate or correct in other situations.
Make sure your answer choice is correct for the case/scenario presented.

For every test question: Take about 10 seconds or so to ask some of the following:

Which information is correct in the question?
Which ones are possible distractors?
What are the assumptions made in the question?
Are the various information stated in the question consistent or inconsistent?
Which one of the information is the priority action?
Which one is very relevant for the patient at the specific time, in the specific patient setting?

13: In multiple choice questions, two or three of the options may all be correct. Your job is to choose the most correct, the best correct answer for a particular or specific scenario.

14: Look for the odd options, they may be unrelated to the stem or may not be correct for the particular case scenario. At other times, an answer option that is different from all the others may actually prove to be the correct answer choice.

15: Look for important details about the client or the problem, see if those details are relevant to the client situation or the problem presented.

16: When a question is asking for a negative or false statement, make a note of that, so you don't give a positive answer where a negative answer is required and vice versa.

17: When one part of an answer is wrong, the whole answer may be wrong, and vice versa.

18: When there are two answer choices that have opposites, example: Constipation or diarrhea, urinary hesitancy or urinary urgency, tachycardia or bradycardia, high temperatures or cold temperatures, one of the choices may be the correct answer. Your job is to know which one that is.

19: When two answers seem correct, compare and contrast their differences, there may be just a slight variation that will make one answer more correct than the other.
Select the answer that is most prudent, most logical, most safe, most priority in your best clinical judgment.

20: Treat the Select All That Applies (SATA) questions as True and False Questions

21: Remember: Sometimes, the longest answer options may be the correct answer.

22: When a situation has equipment failure versus patient, choose patient over equipment. Assess the patient first before checking the equipment.

23: Know what nursing action to implement first in any particular patient situation?
Know what the **priority** nursing intervention is in the answer options.

24: Use the Global, the Umbrella Principle:
If all the answer options appear to be correct, and one answer options seem to include all or most of the ideas of the other answer options, then choose that one. **The all-inclusive, the all-**

encompassing, the global, the umbrella option may be the correct answer, if it includes the ideas or concepts for some or all of the other answer choices.

25: The following are parts of exam questions: The case/scenario, the stem, the correct response and the distractors. When you look at a case scenario, understand the various parts of the question. Look at the part that specifically asks the question: **The STEM.**

26: Pay particular attention to the STEM:

The **Stem** is the part of the statement that explains the issue or asks the question. It is the part of the question that has information about a clinical or pathophysiological issue. The Stem may be keywords or phrases that explain what the purpose of the question is.

In multiple choice questions the STEM is the part that explains the problem or the case, and then there are the answer options consisting of "the CORRECT answer and the "DISTRACTORS" which are the "WRONG" answers

The **STEM** contains very important clues about the main idea or theme of the question that could guide you to choose the right answer choice. Make sure each answer choice has a connection to the Stem.

If the Stem has a positive context, the related answer may be one that is true. A negatively worded Stem may be related to a false idea: a negative answer.

A Stem may be requesting either a negative or a positive response to the answer.

Stems are worded in different formats. Stems may be written as complete or incomplete sentences, others may be written in question formats.

The Stem may have information about some nursing action or a nursing duty like patient teaching.

Remember: Pay very close attention to the Stem. Understand what the Stem is looking for before you choose your answer. Know who and what the question is talking about or focused on. Understand the issue presented in the stem. Ask what is wrong, why it is wrong and know who is affected.

After reading a question /scenario, re-state the question in your own words to help you understand what the question or the stem is really asking you to do. Know the Key Concepts or ideas presented in the stem
Watch for reliability of the information presented in the question VS. the answer choice.

Watch for gaps or discrepancies.

Watch for inconsistency in grammar between the stem and the answer choices.

Watch for commonalities and differences.

Understand what is happening. **Understand what the question is asking.**
See if you can come up with your answer in your head, before looking at the given answer options. See if your answer matches any of the given options.
Look at situations in a holistic manner.
Know what the nurse is being asked to do. **Know which nursing action is priority.**

With each test question, quickly ask yourself: Are there any clusters? any common ideas? Any differences? Any relationships in the information or data given in the questions?

Choose answers that are most GLOBAL, choose answers that show the most "PRIORITY interventions for the patient or the individual presented in the Stem or Question.

Visualize, analyze the correctness of the situations. Choose answer options that maintain physiologic integrity, safe, caring, psychosocial integrity and maximize or promote health. Disregard unrelated facts; be sure you have good rationales for your answers choices.

27: The ABSOLUTES: Take Note of ABSOLUTES, these Words usually point to the wrong answers.
They are Words like **ALWAYS, NEVER, NONE, ONLY, ALL, EVERY, NEVER, NOTHING, TOTAL and so on**

Be very careful with these words. In nursing care, as in life, there are usually some exceptions to most things. The correct test answers are usually not very restrictive.

28: The KEYWORDS: Take Note of KEYWORDS

It is very important to Identify and understand the KEYWORDS in all test questions.

Examples of keywords include: (On admission, Common, Most common, Less common, Best, Least, Not, Is, Initially, Initial response, Best response, Initial action, First, First response, Earliest, Immediately, Highest Priority, First Priority, Most important, Best, Most, Essential, Immediate, Last, Least, Not, Except, Late sign, Early sign and so on.)

These **KEYWORDS may** help you focus and direct your attention to what the question is actually about.
 KEYWORDS may show relationship between the question and the right answer:
Keywords may show relationships between the client, the problem, and the possible correct solutions.

Look for KEYWORDS; **take note of Keywords in the questions,**

29: DISTRACTORS: Watch out for the DISTRACTORS:

Be aware of answer options that repeat the same ideas but in a different wording. These answer choices may mean the same thing but are just restated in different wording, so as to act as distractors or decoys in the given answer choices.

Watch out for answer choices that use synonyms, from one option to the other, they may just be distractors.

Eliminate the easy to identify wrong answers, disregard the obvious wrong answer, before choosing the BEST right answer.

Eliminate obvious distractors. Don't be distracted by the "DISTRACTING DECOYS" find the one correct answer among the DECOYS. Your JOB in the exam is to choose the ONE CORRECT answer among the several decoys or WRONG answers.

30: DIFFICULT QUESTIONS: No one knows everything.
If a question appears very difficult, don't waste too much time on it. Make the best-educated guesses to answer these questions.
Write the numbers of the difficult question on the scratch paper and continue with the exam. Move on, don't linger around on difficult questions, move on to the next question.
If possible come back and Review the skipped questions at the end of the test.
During the exam, you may be lucky to come across similar scenarios or answer choices that may give you clues, about correct answers to difficult questions that you had seen earlier in the exam.

31: As you review to understand each question, allocate appropriate time to each individual question. Do not waste too much time on any individual question.
Focus on each individual questions at hand.
Answer all questions as you go through the exam.
Remember, do not skip any questions.
Again, write the numbers of the "difficult questions" down on the scratch paper.

Complete the whole test, then if you can, come back to recheck the "difficult questions" when you review the completed test.

32: As much as you can, try to **Clarify, Verify, Justify** the correctness of your decisions for all of your answer choices.
Have a working rationale in your head for each individual answer choice.

Choose the answer that makes the most sense in your critical, best nursing judgment. Choose the answer that maximizes patient outcomes the most. Choose the most priority option, the safest and the most global answer options.

Choose the best correct answers using critical thinking, and safe nursing judgments. Choose the answer that is most correct in the setting of the question you are presently looking at.

Do not second guess yourself. If you have done all of the above, then **avoid changing your answer choices.**

Remember: Change your answers only and only if it is absolutely necessary and prudent. Avoid changing your answers.

CHAPTER TEN

Keywords in Sample Practice Questions

1:The word "EXCEPT: "When the keyword **EXCEPT is in the** Stem/the question, this means you have to choose the answer option that is the "Odd Man Out" the choice that is the "Lone man out" the one and only option that is like "an only child" the one that has no relations to the question or the other answer choices or options.

Sample Question:

All of the following agents are used to treat fatigue in MS **Except:**

    A: Methylphenidate
    B: Baclofen
    C: Armodafinil
    D: Modafinil

The correct answer is B: Baclofen. This is the only option that does not belong to the group of medicines used to treat fatigue in MS.
Baclofen is used to treat Spasticity in MS, whereas (Methylphenidate, Armodafinil , and Modafinil) all belong to the group of medications that are used to treat Fatigue in MS.

So in this question, the **"Except"** keyword, refers to the "lone guy out," which in this case is BACLOFEN. Because Baclofen is used to treat spasticity in MS, it has no relations to the other three medications that are used to treat fatigue in MS.

In the Stem/ the Question part here, look at the word **"ALL"**, and the word" **EXCEP**T" to help you know what the question is asking. All refers to the three agents: (Methylphenidate,

Armodafinil, and Modafinil) **Except** refers to the single agent, (Baclofen)

So the keyword is **EXCEPT** in the **Stem** of the question means, you are being asked to single out, leave out, omit, the option that has no relation to the other answer choices or the question at hand.

2: The Keyword "**NOT**"

The key word "**NOT**" in the Stem or the Question, means you are being asked to choose the answer option that is unrelated to all the other choices, the one that is the odd one out, that is NOT connected or related to the question or the other answer choices, the one that is not correct, the one that has the wrong connection to the question or answer options.

Example:

Which of the following statements about Multiple Sclerosis (MS) is **NOT** correct?

A: MS is an autoimmune, immune-mediated, inflammatory disease
B: MS is a demyelinating disorder of the Central Nervous System
C: MS is more prevalent in people of African American descent
D: MS is the most common neurological disorder that affects young adults.

Option C is the correct answer here. Based on the pathophysiology and demographics of MS, options A, B and D are all true statements about the disease, option C is not.

Note: The use of the keywords EXCEPT and NOT in the STEM or Question are kind of synonymous or similar. They both require you to choose an option that has no connection to the stem or the other answer choices presented. They point to the answer choice

43

that does not fit the case scenario or subject matter presented in the stem.

Here you are required to look at the keyword (Except or Not) in the stem/question, determine the relationships, then choose the correct answer option.

3: The Key Word " **PRIMARY"** means you are being asked to choose the answer option that is the main cause of an issue, the root cause of something, the chief reason why something is happening, the first, the principal, the fundamental reason why a disease process or condition occurred. You are being asked to choose the reason why something happened in the first place. The main reason, the etiology or root cause of an abnormality of some sort.

Example:

Which of the following is a **Primary** cause of cognitive changes in Multiple Sclerosis?

- A: Depression
- B: Fatigue
- C: Stress
- D: Axonal damage

The **correct answer is D:** Axonal damage. As the demyelination, nerve cell and axonal damage occur in MS, the conduction of impulses in the brain is impacted. Depression, Fatigue, and stress are all SECONDARY causes of cognitive changes.

The depression, fatigue and stress all occurred from secondary effects of the MS, which was caused by axonal damage in the first place. Depression and the other problems are the "sequela", the secondary or after effect of the MS disease. The axonal damage in the CNS is the first cause of the problem of the cognitive changes.

Note: "SECONDARY" which is the opposite "PRIMARY" can also be used as a keyword.

4: When the keyword "LEAST" is seen in a question, it means, choose the option that has the smallest effect, the lowest relevance or importance, the one that is the smallest in size, degree or amount. The one that has the lowest impact or importance in a given situation or scenario.

Example:

The **least** likely cognitive function affected in MS is:

A: Long-Term memory
B: Short-Term Memory
C: Problem solving and abstract reasoning
D: Concentration and attention

The **correct answer is "A."** In MS, events that occurred "long ago" in the distant past, ones that are stored in the long-term memory, can remain intact longer. The other cognitive abilities tend to deteriorate more. The cognitive ability that is affected the lowest, the smallest; the least is the Long-Term memory.

The opposite of the Key Word LEAST is" MOST"
The Keyword MOST in the Stem or Question requires you to choose the option that has the highest significance, the highest amount or quantity, or the one that has the highest effect or degree of impact on a problem or case presented in the question or the Stem.

In general, The Keywords: MOST Essential, INITIAL response, FIRST Response, IMMEDIATE are all asking you to choose the Highest Priority, the Most Significant, the Top option amongst a group of answer choices that are comparably all good or correct. The Immediate, the initial responses are the highest class, the very best option out of all the other good answers or options. You are asked to choose the PRIORITY option, the one that will have the BEST patient outcome, one that has the MOST benefit for the patient. It requires one to choose the most correct, the most significant, the most priority, the FIRST out of the other correct answer options, the one that is the best choice out of the other given correct options.

When you see these keywords, think" MASLOW" think PRIORITY, think the BEST, First action to implement. That means the most significant, best option. Here you are required to choose the Number One nursing action, amongst other relatively good options in the presented case, situation or scenario.

When you see the Keywords: "is CORRECT" "NOT CORRECT", "TRUE", "IS NOT TRUE" Basically these keywords in the stem or question are the same as "TRUE/FALSE," questions. You are being asked to distinguish facts/true from "untrue" items. You are required to separate the true statement from the false statements or vice versa.

If the question or the stem is: Which of the following is "NOT CORRECT"
Then look for the "false" the negative, the untrue option in the presented answer choices.
Be careful not to choose a positive or true answer option when you are required to choose the negative option that relates to the stem, the case scenario presented and vice versa .

When you see the keyword: ANALYZE: It means to look at a concept or statement in detail, take it apart, examine its various parts in a logical and methodical manner, look for the root cause, interrelationships, and make criticisms or conclusions. Break the issue apart, using supportive arguments and evidence for and against your conclusions or decisions

The Keyword EVALUATE: Means to describe, explain, analyze the result of some action, make informed judgements, verdict or conclusion about the results. Make decisions for or against an action, an event using supportive evidence to justify your conclusions. In patient's situations you evaluate your nursing interventions or actions to determine if they had positive or negative results.

When you see the keyword ASSESS or ASSESSMENT: It means you look at an issue, a patient or some situation, paying attentions to positive or negative results or aspects that can have important contributions to other processes. You examine patients, and then use the noticeable evidence or data to make informed judgments, decisions, and conclusions about causes or findings in patient situations.

Example:

5: You are performing an initial assessment on your MS patient at the hospital, as you firmly stroke the sole of her foot, you notice dorsiflexion of her big toe, while her other toes fan outwards.
You interpret this finding as a:

    A: Negative Babinski response
    B: Positive Babinski response
    C: Positive Romberg test
    D: A negative Romberg test

The correct answer is B: The big toe extends upwards/dorsiflexes, the other toes fan outwards, as pressure is applied to the lateral aspect of the sole of the foot during assessment/examination.

A Positive Barbinski sign indicates an abnormality in the motor control pathways of the CNS.

The Romberg Test looks for balance and proprioception defects.
The patient stands with her feet together and her eyes closed, while her balance and posture are assessed by the health care professional.

CHAPTER ELEVEN

Some Test Taking Tips to Remember

REMEMBER: CRITICAL THINKING, THINK NURSING PROCESS, THINK BLOOMS TAXONOMY
(from lowest to highest, PRIORITIZE)

REMEMBER: In certification exams, some of the assigned questions may be pretest/sample questions for future tests, they may not be scored. Regardless of that fact, treat every question with the utmost seriousness. You won't know the few questions that are not counted in your exam. As the exam candidate, in your eyes, every question is important and critical.

REMEMBER: As you proceed through this exam, do not leave any question unanswered. **Answer all questions.** During the exam, mark, write down the question number of the answer choices you are not sure about. If allowed, If you have time left, come back to them, when you review the whole exam before the test ends.

REMEMBER: Unless you are absolutely confident that you have very good rationales to do so, do not be in the habit of changing your answers.

REMEMBER: Choose the answer that is the most significant, that is the most Priority and the safest for the patient in the particular situation, setting or case scenario.

Watch for stressors in patient situations. As you choose your answers, eliminate stressors and risks that will compromise patient safety and patient outcomes.

Again, REMEMBER: When you get your scratch paper at the Exam site, quickly:

DO a "BRAIN DUMP" right away!

Take a minute or two to quickly write down important Acronyms, Mnemonics, and any short-hand information that can quickly trigger your memory to recall important concepts, content or ideas during the exam.

You are simply doing a quick "unloading" of important facts from your brain to the scratch paper. During the test, you could use this information as a "quick reference tool" to trigger your memory, to help recall information faster, if the need ever arises.

CHAPTER TWELVE

When in Doubt

REMEMBER the Following:
The Nursing Process
Maslow's Hierarchy of Needs
The ABCs in patient care
Patient Safety, Patient's Right, Patient's privacy
Nursing Delegation,
Therapeutic Communication, Psychosocial needs of patients
Kubler-Ross's Stages of Grief and other nursing theories and concepts.
Use Critical thinking.
Think Priority, think patient safety, and think about the best outcome for patients

Remember, in situations where therapeutic communication is required, always acknowledge and validate patient's feelings before you give information. The patient is the focus and center in nursing care.

In multiple choice questions, if three of the choices are similar, then the one option that is different may be the correct answer.

If two of the answer choices say the same exact thing or give the same or similar information, then usually both options may be wrong.

Select the "UMBRELLA OPTION" The "GLOBAL" The most comprehensive, the one that provides or addresses the most needs, the most effective multiple ways of resolving the issue presented in the question.

REMEMBER: Pace yourself well. Manage your test time well. Do not run out of time before answering all 150 questions.

ANSWER ALL QUESTIONS!

Comprehension of required content, Good study techniques and knowledge of critical test taking skills can be some of the best arsenals to help one pass the MSCN examination.

> Get plenty of sleep the night before the exams.
> On your exam day, have a protein bar or some kind of healthy snack handy.
> Find the exam site and get there early.
> Good preparation will help reduce anxiety on the test date.

Be Confident! If you have studied well and given it your all,
BE CONFIDENT!

Envision yourself PASSING the EXAM.
Envision the MSCN credentials at the end of your name!

Take some Deep Breaths,
Go on, Go take the test, you got this.
Go Get Your MSCN Certification!!!

CHAPTER THIRTEEN

Some Benefits of Certification

Professional specialty certifications have both personal and professional benefits.

Being certified brings a sense of accomplishment, fulfillment, confidence and pride.

Certified nurses are respected among their peers.

Certification shows a higher level of competence, adds credence and validation of a nurse's clinical knowledge and professional competence among their peers.
Supervisors, administrators and patients recognize a certified nurse as one who is more knowledgeable and much more clinically competent.

As part of maintaining their certification credentials, Certified Nurses can be much more committed to lifelong learning and continuing education. Required continuing education keeps the certified nurse much more abreast of current evidenced-based knowledge and information in their chosen specialty area.

Preparation and studying for certification require knowledge of core critical nursing information in the specific specialty areas.
Nurses who have prepared well and successfully complete such exams gain invaluable clinical knowledge that can translate to improved nursing care in the specific patient care settings.

Certified Nurses have improved confidence and personal satisfactions.
In some clinical settings, certified nurses are paid more than their peers who are not certified.

Certified Nurses may have better job and professional advancement opportunities than the non-certified nurses.

CONCLUSION

There is no doubt the Multiple Sclerosis Nursing International Certification Examination can be challenging.

Certification examinations as a whole require good preparation and some form of commitment from candidates who aspire to pass these exams. A combination of good study techniques and knowledge of critical test taking skills can be some of the best arsenals to help one pass nursing certification examinations in general.

Preparing and studying for the MSCN exams require a lot of hard work and commitment on your part. I personally had to count on hard work, some solid test preparation strategies and test-taking techniques to help me PASS my MSCN Exam, at the very First Attempt.

As a nurse, your success in passing this exam may bring you personal and professional benefits, but most importantly though, the patients you care for will have a certified nurse who has gained invaluable critical knowledge that can translate into better patient outcomes.

You are a nurse; your patients' care and safety depend on your clinical knowledge, your expertise, competence, dedication and compassion.

Do yourself and your patients a big favor, strive to be the best always. Get Certified!

Plan well. Do what needs to be done. Leave no stone unturned. Give it your all!

Believe in yourself! Be Confident! You are a Nurse! You got this! Go for it! Get Certified!

Nurses are life-long learners. Our patients depend and count on our expertise and knowledge as we provide care in our various clinical settings. We can all benefit from learning from one another.

If you have any advice or suggestions that other colleagues can benefit from, please feel free to notify me.

My contact information is: **adayans@gmail.com** or **info@elitecarecorp.com**

Thank you for reading my book!

GOOD LUCK!

Appendix A : Multiple Sclerosis Disease Modifying Medications

Injectable Medications

Rebif   (interferon beta-1a)

Avonex (interferon beta-1a)

Plegridy (Peginterferon beta-1a)

Rebif, Avonex, and Plegridy are interferon beta-1a *(M*nemonic: RAP)

Betaseron

Extavia Betaseron and Extavia are both Interferon beta-1b

(Mnemonic: BE) 1b

Glatopa (Glatiramer acetate) is the generic version of Copaxone 20 mg dose.

Copaxone (Glatiramer acetate) Copaxone comes in 20mg and 40mg doses.

ZINBRYTA (Daclizumab) : FDA approved for Multiple Sclerosis treatment in May 2016.

<u>Oral Medications</u>

Tecfidera (Dimethyl fumarate)

Aubagio (Teriflunomide)

Gilenya (Fingolimod)

Oral disease modifying agents —-   Mnemonic:- (*TAG*)

Intravenous Medications

Lemtrada   (Alemtuzumab)

Novantrone (Mitoxantrone)

Tysabri (Natalizumab)

LiNT,silent i,for IV meds. reminder, or **MAN** for **M**itoxantrone, **A**lemtuzumab, **N**atalizumab.

Appendix: B Online Resources

Multiple Sclerosis Nurses International Certification Board: http://www.msnicb.org

Professional Testing Corporation (PTC)
www.ptcny.com

International Organization of Multiple Sclerosis Nurses:
http://www.iomsn.org

Consortium of Multiple Sclerosis Centers:
http://www.mscare.org

MS Views and News: http://www.msviews.org

National Multiple Sclerosis Society (NMSS)
http://www.nmss.org

Multiple Sclerosis Association of America (MSAA)
http://www.msaa.com

Multiple Sclerosis International Federation:
http://www.msif.org

Multiple Sclerosis Foundation (MSF)
http://www.msfocus.org

Multiple Sclerosis Awareness Foundation (MSAF):
http://www.msawareness.org

Can Do Multiple Sclerosis: http://www.mscando.org

The Myelin Project USA: http://www.myelin.org

MS World: http://www.msworld.org

Appendix: C Pharmaceutical Companies

Teva (Glatiramer Acetate/ Copaxone): www.copaxone.com

Serono (Rebif): http://mslifelines.com

Accorda (Dalfampradine; Ampyra): http://www.ampyra.com

Novatis (Extavia; Interferon beta-1b; Fingolimod/ Gilenya): http://www.extavia.com

Sanofi Genzyme (alentuzumab/ Lemtrada): http://www.lemtrada.com

Genzyme: (Teriflunomide/Aubagio): http://www.aubagio.com

Biogen (1. Natalizumab/Tysabri. 2. Dymethylfumarate / Tecfidera)

References

Halper, June., & Harris Colleen. (2012). Nursing Practice in Multiple Sclerosis: A Core Curriculum (3rd Ed). New York, NY: Springer Publishing Company

Halper, June., & Holland, N. J. (2011). Comprehensive Nursing Care In Multiple Sclerosis (3rd Ed). New York, NY: Springer Publishing Company

Birnbaum, G. L. (2013). Multiple Sclerosis: Clinician's Guide to Diagnosis and Treatment
New York, NY: Oxford University Press

Macaluso, V. F. (2015). Multiple Sclerosis From Both Sides of the Desk
Bloomington, IN: IUniverse

American Association of Critical-Care Nurses (AACN). (2015). Homepage
Retrieve from http://www.aacn.org

Bloom's Taxonomy (2016). Homepage
Retrieved from: www.bloomstaxonomy.org

Brorsen, A.J., & Rogelet, K.R (2014). Adult CCRN Certification Review
Burlington, MA: Jones & Bartlett Learning.

Sheremata, W. A. (2011).100 Questions & Answers About Multiple Sclerosis (2nd Ed.)
Sudbury, MA: Jones & Bartlett Learning.

www.ingramcontent.com/pod-product-compliance
Lightning Source LLC
Chambersburg PA
CBHW070257290326
41930CB00041B/2632